A Nurse's Recipe Book for Patient Care

A Basic Guide for Nursing Students, New Nurses and Nurses who are working in a Hospital

I would like to dedicate this book to all of the nursing students and nurses that I have taught over the years.

I would also like to dedicate this book to Rachael and Kim. You guys are great!

I would also like to dedicate this book to Veronica.

Please Read

First, I need to say that this book is not meant to diagnose or dictate the care received for anyone. It is simply a guide for common care not specialized care. Every patient is different and the care is based on the patient. This book is meant as a guide for nurses.

With that all said, I can begin talking with you. When I was a new nurse, I had no idea that many common patient problems had treatment algorithms. It took me years to learn these. Some are based on medical regulations, while others are based on acute care practice.

I am writing this book as a request from many students over the years. When I teach, I compare medical treatment to recipes. If you were going to make a brownie, you would use certain ingredients. If you were going to make lasagna, you would also use certain ingredients. Most of the time, basic medical treatment is the same way. When we have pneumonia, there is a certain treatment path that we often follow. When we are treating a-fib, there is also a specific path that we follow. This book is a basic attempt to simplify the basic care that many patients receive. My promise to you is that I will try my best to make it as simple as possible. Just remember that this is a basic guide, not a medical guide. It is not meant to diagnose- MD's do that part. Okay let's start.

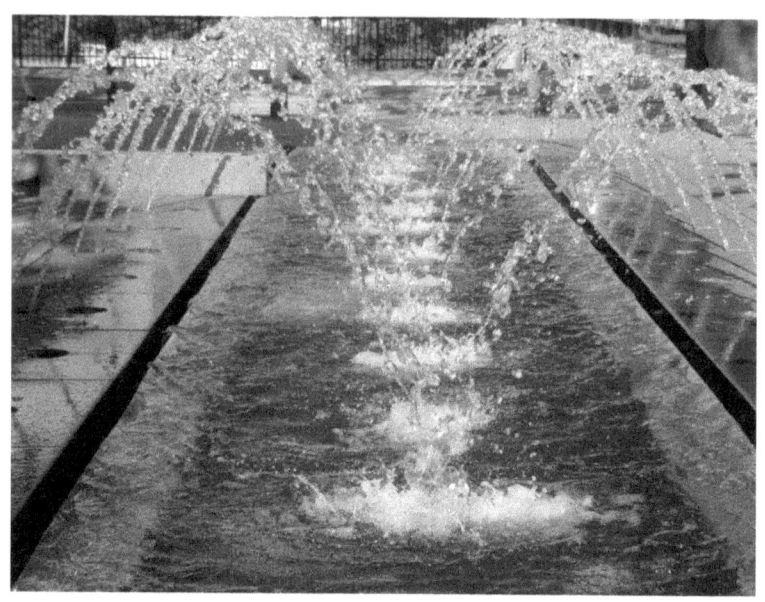

"Be the change you want to see in the world. "

~Mohandas Gandhi

Points to remember

Doctors diagnose diseases (DDD), nurses do not (NDN). We are the ones who care for the patients and report changes in symptoms. Although we know that it may "look like a duck and quack like a duck," we cannot say that it is a duck because it may be a goose. Finding out that it is a goose or a duck takes tests and knowledge. Finding out that it is a goose or a duck is the medical doctor's job.

Your job as an acute care nurse is to monitor the changes. If there is a change in patient condition, you have several options:

1. You can call the doctor.
2. You can call respiratory STAT.
3. You can call the charge nurse for help and advice.
4. You can call the rapid response team or the medical emergency team (same thing, different name).
5. You can call a code.
6. You can jump around and panic- although this is not advised and will not help the patient.

   If you are taking any of the above steps, you should let your charge nurse know that something is going wrong with the patient. This is a common courtesy and you may need help. It is also known as escalating the chain of command and helps you cover yourself. On the same note, calling you charge nurse will not help the patient in itself. You need to take other actions. He/she is there for advice and assistance. If there is time, you can call the doctor. If time is not on your side and the patient is appearing unstable, call a rapid medical team. It is easy as that.

Time Management is the Key

Being a nurse can be challenging. Most of the time you are responsible for the care of multiple patients. Each one deserves your time, however there is only one of you. You have to learn to divide your time evenly between all of the patients and the other tasks that need to be done (like charting). This is why it is so important that nurses learn to utilize their resources. When you are in the hospital, you have an entire team that can help. Some of the members of the team may include:

- Your patient care technicians
- Your charge nurse
- Your nursing supervisor
- Respiratory therapists
- Resource nurse
- Other nurses
- Security
- Chaplains
- Medical staff

There are probably more team members are available, however this is the basics. The point is **time management is the key.** You only have so much time. You may have 4 or more patients and EACH ONE DESERVES YOUR TIME. You cannot stay in any one room for too long of a period without checking in with all of your other patients.

This is probably one of the biggest issue that I see with newer nurses. Yes, we all want to provide the best care for each of our patients, however when you give too much time to one patient, the others suffer. All of your patients are in the hospital because they do not feel well. You have to care for each of them and chart your care. Time is important.

Charting and Record Keeping

When you are a nurse, charting is essential. It is the thing that will help keep you from being sued or getting in trouble with the hospital. You have to keep track of what you did and when you did it. I can't even begin to highlight the importance of charting.

You probably heard the saying, "If you did not chart it, you did not do it." Charting is one of the only ways that you have to show that you took action. It is there to protect you and the patient.

A few pointers on charting:

- Chart as close to real time as you can. This shows that you are watching the patient and monitoring changes.
- Be accurate. If you did it, chart it.
- If you see changes in a patient's condition, take action and then chart it.
- If your hospital has a medication scanner, make sure that you use it.
- Documentation is the primary way that all practitioners can communicate with each other.
- Your charting can mean the difference of the hospital being reimbursed for services from insurance companies including Medicare/Medicaid.
- The electronic and paper chart is a legal document.
- Failure to document can be interpreted as neglect. Always chart the care you provide.
- Use the patient's own words when possible.
- Chart what you do and what you see. Do not make assumptions.

- Nursing notes should be consistent with the rest of the charting. Don't contradict yourself.
- Always chart when you talk with a doctor about a patient's concerns or care. If you inform a doctor of something, chart it.
- Always make sure that your actions and charting are consistent with the hospital policies and procedures.

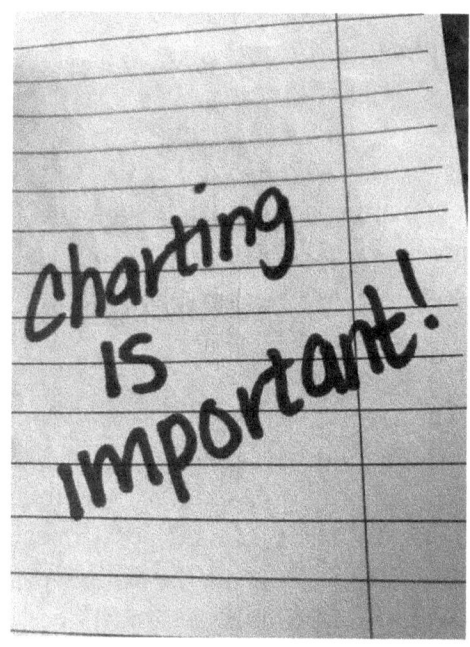

Hospital Policy

Every hospital has policies that guide care and help the nurses make decisions. Many professionals contribute to the creation of the policies. In fact, many hospitals have committees that work on the policies.

Hospital nursing policies protect the hospital, the patient and the nurse. As long as you are abiding by the policies, you will most likely be covered by the hospital if a litigation should arise.

Find out where your hospital policies are and learn them. Many times I will print a copy of the specific policy that I am using and put a paper copy in the front of the chart for reference. For instance if you need to administer a blood product to a patient, find the nursing policy on Blood Administration. Learn the steps that the facility wants you to take when administering blood. Learn what to do if there is an adverse reaction it is okay to print the policy and put it in the front of the chart for reference. If you write a nursing note, you can say, "Administered blood per policy."

Members of the Patient Care Team

There are many professionals that work together to provide care to every patient. It is vital that the nurse know what resources are available on each unit and hospital. Know who you can call for help. And know what their scope of practice is per the policies.

Here is a basic list of the professionals involved in patient care. It is your responsibility to find out what each of the professionals do and if they are available on your unit. A little time for information gathering can really go a long way. Use your resources!

The Patient Care Team

The RN
The LPN
Nursing assistants
Charge nurse (either dedicated or not-dedicated-they either don't have patients or they do).
Other nurses
Respiratory therapists
Occupational therapists
Physical therapists
Nursing supervisor
Nurse manager
Nursing director
Dietary
Lab technicians
Chaplain
Volunteers
Patient transport
Resource nurse
Central supply team
Speech therapy
Pharmacist and pharmacy technicians
Wound nurse
IV team
Nurses from other departments
Cardiac rehab
Social work
Case management
Environmental Services
Maintenance

The Code Cart

The code cart is basically a large metal tool chest on wheels. It is often red and contains emergency medical items. These medical items include everything from emergency medications (no narcotics) to respiratory equipment. Whenever there is a medical emergency, the code cart should be wheeled in the room.

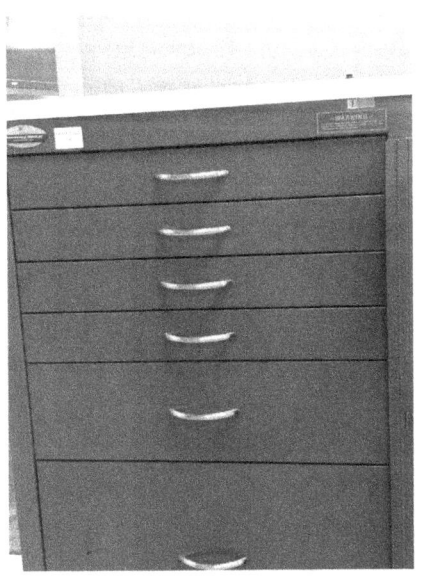

The code cart often contains many medications. Some of these medications often include:

- o Epinephrine (cardiac dose). Remember: THE CART IS FOR THE HEART!
- o Atropine
- o Amiodarone
- o Adenosine
- o Dextrose
- o Narcan
- o Sodium bicarbonate
- o IV bags and tubing (0.9% Normal Saline)
- o Calcium Chloride
- o Dopamine
- o Vasopressin
- o Lidocaine

Most of the medications are usually kept in the first drawer. The other drawers contain intubation equipment such as a bite block, endotracheal tubes, nasopharyngeal airways, laryngoscope handle and blades, stylets, and a bag valve mask (BVM) or (AMBU bag).

IV bags and tubing are also in the crash cart. It is important to know what each drawer contains in your facility. It is also important to know where the code carts are in your unit.

Crash carts should be retrieved any time there is a medical emergency. If a rapid response is called or a code is called, then the cart should be present. The emergency equipment and medications that it contains is vital. In an emergency, time is very valuable.

What the Heck is a Rapid Response Team?

Any time a patient's condition is changing into something that can end badly, a rapid response should be called. Anyone can call a rapid response. This means that a rapid response can be called by a patient, the patient's family, support staff and the nursing staff. A rapid response tells the team that your patient needs help. It gives the nurse extra hands to carry out tasks that need to be carried out fast. Rapid responses save lives.

Rapid response teams may be called medical emergency teams (MET's) or rapid assessment teams (RAT's). When they are called by a nurse, it means that the nurse has sent out a flair. It gives the nurse extra eyes and hands to care for the patient. It allows the nurse to bypass the usual chain of command to get help for the patient. Most rapid response teams have set orders that they are permitted to carry out before they need to call the MD. This saves valuable time that the nurse may need to save a life.

A rapid can be called for many reasons. Some of the reasons include:

> The nurse just has a gut feeling that something is wrong with the patient.
> The patient is showing signs of deterioration
> The patient is having an allergic reaction that is progressing
> The patient needs to be stabilized
> Rapid physiological changes in patient condition

Many nurses have told me that at first, they thought that calling a rapid response meant that they could not handle the situation and it meant that they were a bad nurse. This line of thinking could not be farther from the truth. Summoning the rapid response team means that you care for the patient and want them to have the best care possible. It means that you note that you need extra professionals. It means that you are a great nurse.

There are many people who come to the patient's room when a rapid response is called. Of course the team may vary from hospital to hospital too. Often times, the team may consist of:

- A physician
- Critical care nurse
- Nursing supervisor
- Respiratory therapist
- Clinical specialists

Rapid response teams started back in 2006 when the Institute of Healthcare Improvement (IHI) asked all hospitals to implement this resource. They started the "5 Million Lives Campaign," because the IHI noted that patients often actually start to decline hours before a code is needed.

For more information please visit the IHI at www.IHI.org

Note: When you are going to call a rapid response team, always let your charge nurse know.

Advanced Cardiac Life Support (ACLS)

When I was a new nurse I wondered how nurses knew what to do when a patient coded. I soon found my answer. The American Heart Association has a certification called the Advanced Cardiac Life Support (ACLS) certification. This certification shows medical staff what to do when a patient goes into bradycardia or tachycardia, patients stop breathing, heart rhythm changes and more. The class is offered by most hospitals and is free to the medical staff. The certification is good for 2 years and a renewal class must be taken.

The initial class lasts for 2 days and the renewal class often takes about 5 hours. There is a new trend that allows the medical professional to take the class online with minimal face-to-face instruction. This is a newer way of completing the class.

For more information on the ACLS, please contact the education department in your hospital or visit the American Heart Association at:

https://cpr.heart.org/AHAECC/CPRAndECC/Training/HealthcareProfessional/AdvancedCardiovascularLifeSupportACLS/UCM_473186_Advanced-Cardiovascular-Life-Support-ACLS.jsp

In order to create this book, I asked many of the acute-care nurses I know to identify some of the most common illnesses and conditions they see on a regular basis. These are the conditions that are included in this book.

Patient Care Made Simple:
The Nursing Recipes

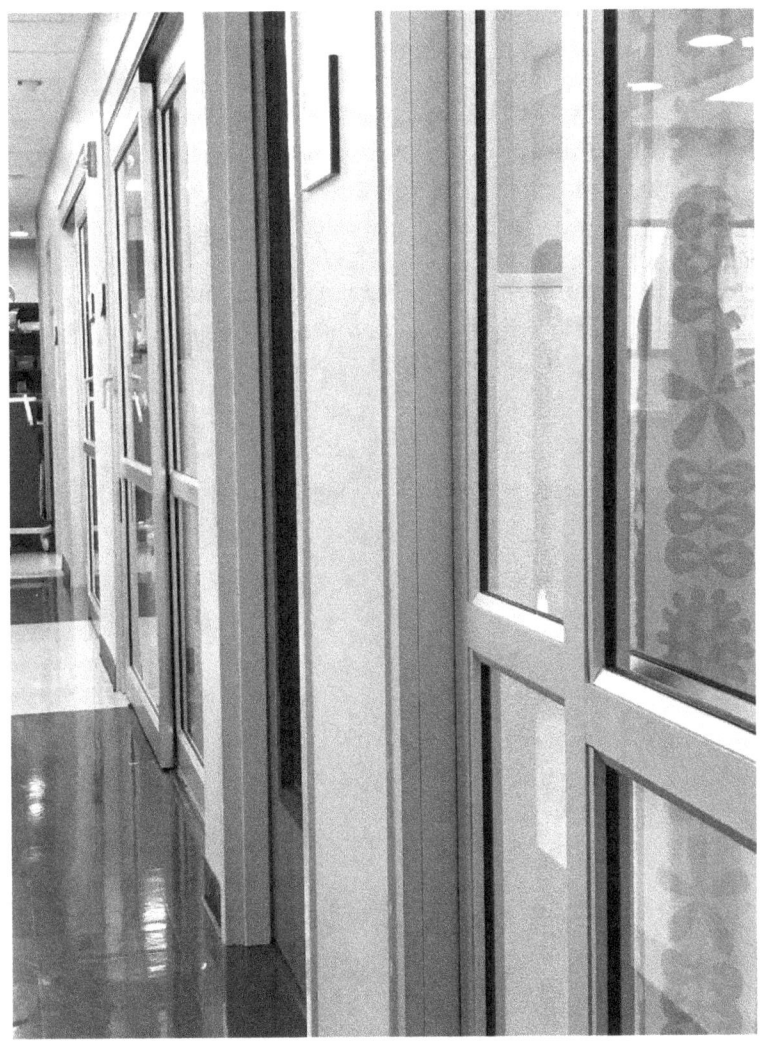

Please take notes on each of the pages. I am leaving plenty of room for you.

Also, remember that these are just the basics. Please consult your hospital policy for specific treatments. Also remember, the physician will tailor the care as he/she sees fit.

These recipes just help the new nurse put things in perspective. As you read through them, please think about WHY the doctor would order these things.

I am not going to review the issues that are covered in the ACLS course.

New Chest Pain

Who are you going to call?

Charge nurse, Rapid response team, physician

The Physician may order:

An EKG (Need to see if it is a STEMI or NSTEMI)
Labs: Cardiac Enzymes, CBC, BMP
Medications: (ONAM)
 Oxygen
 Nitroglycerin (either sublingual, paste or drip)
 Aspirin
 Morphine
Heparin GTT
May also order a GI cocktail

Consult Cardiology
Ultimate goal is often the cath lab
 If it is a STEMI then this has to happen **fast.** If it is a
NSTEMI, the cardiac team can take a little longer.

Atrial Fibrillation with Rapid Ventricular Response
(a-fib w/ RVR)

Goal:

Primary is to reduce the heart rate. Secondary, restore normal sinus rhythm (NSR) if possible.

Who are you going to call?

Charge nurse, Rapid response team, and physician

You need to know:

Vital signs and if the patient is symptomatic (stable or unstable?)

The Physician may order:

An EKG (to verify the rhythm)
Labs: Cardiac Enzymes, CBC, BMP
Cardizem bolus and drip
    Or Amiodarone drip
Pt may need O2

Consult Cardiology

The primary goal is to slow the heart down. The secondary goal is to get the patient back into normal sinus rhythm. While the cardiologist tries to get the patient back into normal sinus rhythm, he/she may order anticoagulants to help prevent blood clots from forming.

If the medications do not work to get the heart back into normal sinus rhythm (NSR), or if the patient is not stable, the cardiologist may try cardioversion or, as a last resort, ablation.

Treating New Pneumonia

Diagnose:

Chest X-ray (possibly daily)
ABG's
Sputum Culture
Blood Culture
Possible flu culture and other respiratory cultures

Medications/Checkpoints:

The Physician may order:

0.9% NS Fluid Bolus followed by fluids (unless they have CHF)
Broad spectrum IV antibiotic (until sputum culture results are received, then the antibiotic will be more specific)
> Nurse must review patient allergies before the administration of antibiotics.
> Monitor the patient while infusing IV antibiotics
> As patient improves, antibiotics will change from IV to PO

Guaifenesin
Acetaminophen
Encourage Incentive spirometer use while the patient is in bed
O2 as needed
A Pulmonology MD may be consulted to assist in managing care
If your patient is not in the ICU, a continuous pulse ox may be a great idea (In the ICU everyone gets a pulse ox automatically).
Monitor signs/symptoms
Provide your patient with tissues and a quiet environment

Possible Sepsis

Diagnose:

Chest X-ray, UA
ABG's
Sputum Culture
Blood Culture
Possible flu culture and other respiratory cultures

Medications/Checkpoints:

The Physician may order:

Fluid Bolus followed by fluids (unless they have CHF)
    Initial fluid bolus is usually 30 ml/kg
    Must support the blood pressure!
Once blood culture is collected, start Broad spectrum IV
        antibiotics (until sputum culture results are
        received, then the antibiotic will be more specific),
        may also start antifungals and antiviral medications
        Nurse must review patient allergies before the
        administration of antibiotics.
Monitor the patient while infusing IV antibiotics
As patient improves, antibiotics will change from IV to PO
Guaifenesin
Acetaminophen
Encourage Incentive spirometer use while the patient is in
        Bed

Monitor vital signs, patient condition and assess regularly.

The Review of the Sepsis Train

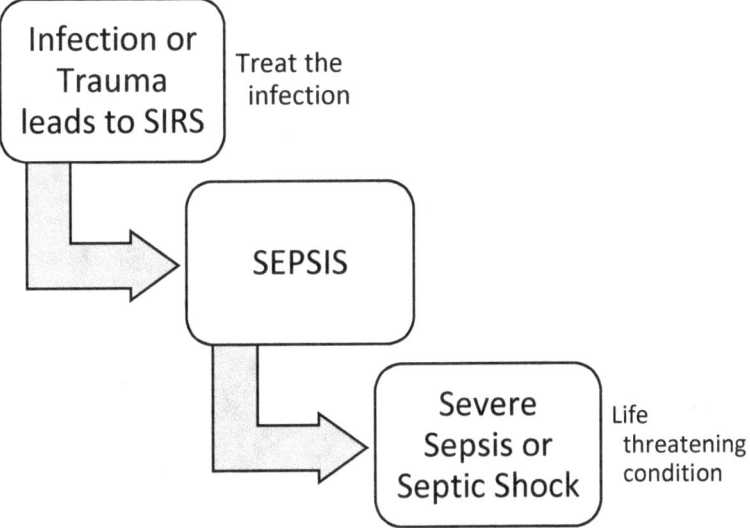

Infection or Trauma leads to SIRS — Treat the infection

SEPSIS

Severe Sepsis or Septic Shock — Life threatening condition

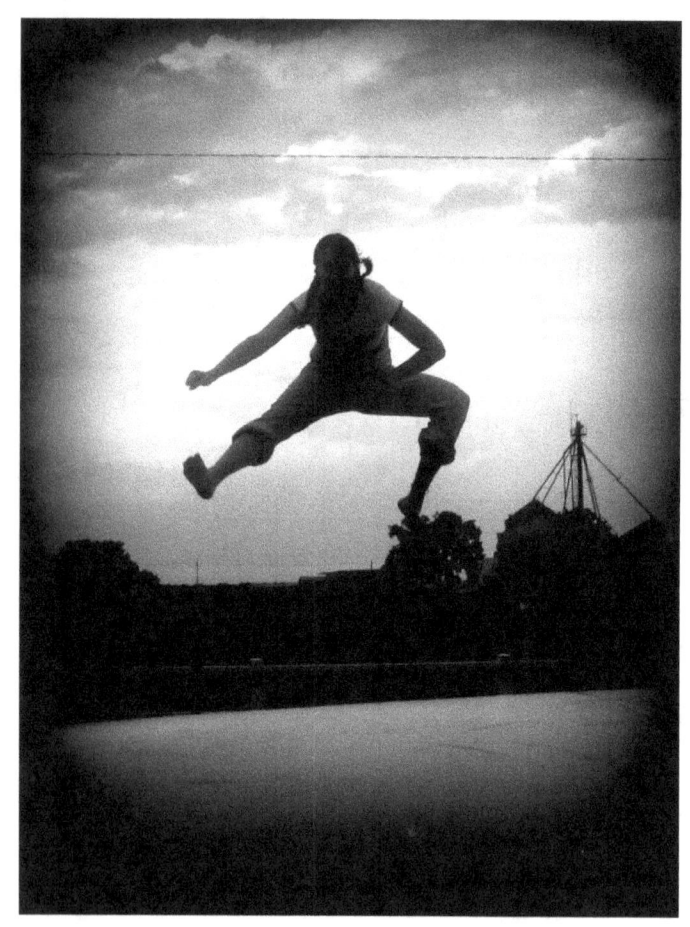

Let's Talk about O2 Assistance

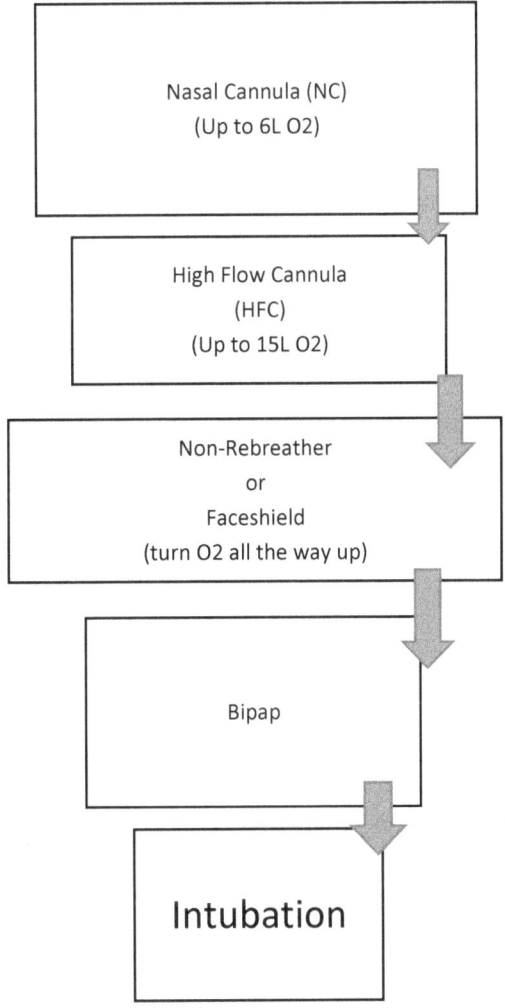

Nasal Cannula (NC)
(Up to 6L O2)

High Flow Cannula
(HFC)
(Up to 15L O2)

Non-Rebreather
or
Faceshield
(turn O2 all the way up)

Bipap

Intubation

ECMO

If the heart and lungs need to rest, then the only option left is Extracorporeal Membrane Oxygenation (ECMO) also called heart-lung bypass. ECMO is a very expensive and complicated process. It literally is a machine that is able to circulate the blood and add oxygen. It is always done in the ICU and only a few hospitals in each area are able to perform this treatment.

I remember the first time I ever saw a person on ECMO. I was a nursing student and amazed at the process. The patient is not able to leave the hospital room because they are attached to the machine, which can be difficult for a younger person. The person that I saw on ECMO was waiting on a heart transplant and knew that this was the only way to stay alive.

The ECMO rooms almost always have reverse isolation precautions. These patients have an increase in their infection risks and must be protected at all costs. In fact, hospitals who perform ECMO often have a special room that is dedicated to the process.

ECMO can be performed on most people. It can also be performed on babies. Just remember that it is the last medical effort that we have available and only a few hospitals have the resources to perform it.

Allergic Reaction

Anaphylaxis

Who are you going to call?

  Charge nurse, Rapid response team, and physician

First stop the cause if possible

The physician may order:

0.1 to 0.3 mg of Epinephrine (1:1,000) IM

IV steroid (Solu-Medrol)
Diphenhydramine IV
0.9% Normal Saline bolus

*If the blood pressure is low the physician may order catecholamines (dopamine, norepinephrine, epinephrine, etc.)

*The physician may order albuterol to help with bronchospasms.

It is important to:

Monitor vital signs and patient condition

Protect the airway

Patient may need to be flat in bed with legs elevated to keep blood circulating to the brain.

Overdose

Opiate Overdose

Naloxone (Narcan or Evzio)
Supportive care

Points to remember:

- Must repeat dose as needed as the antidote only lasts a few minutes.
- Go low, start slow.
- People can wake up punching after administration-the medication shocks the system.
- Any overdose can be very dangerous, however it is even more dangerous when people mix drugs or the drugs contain additives. For instance if someone mixes cocaine and heroin, if medical professionals reverse the heroin, the cocaine overdose takes over. Be prepared for anything.

- *For an interesting story about a fatal combination overdose, look up information/videos about River Phoenix's fatal overdose at Johnny Depp's nightclub, called The Viper Room, located in Los Angeles, California.*

Benzodiazepine Overdose

Flumazenil
Supportive Care

Seizures

Goal:
Protect the patient during the seizure.
Stop seizure if necessary.

Who do you call?
Charge nurse, rapid response, and physician

You Need to Know:

- Turn the patient on his/her side.
- Do not place anything in the patient's mouth.
- Implement seizure precautions
- Note the characteristics of the seizure
- Note the duration of the seizure
- Protect the airway
- Monitor vital signs
- Suction as needed
- Apply O2 as indicated

The physician may order:

- Ativan or another benzo to stop the seizure if it lasts beyond 3-5 minutes or is recurring.
- Longer term IV seizure medications like Levetracetam (Keppra) or Valproic Acid
- EEG
- STAT CT scan

Violent Patient

Goal:
To keep the patient and staff safe.

Who do you call?
Security, charge nurse, rapid response

You need to know:

- The most important thing is to keep everyone safe. First we need to keep the staff safe and then the patient. Do not put yourself in a compromising situation.
- Activate a Code Green (or whatever color your facility has assigned). Let security deal with the violence. They are trained to deal with this.
- Know that you may have to sedate and restrain your patient.
- It is important to figure out the cause of the agitation

The physician may order:

- Restraints
- Sedatives
- STAT CT
- MRI
- Blood gases
- Labs

Alcohol Withdrawal

Goal:

Keep patient and staff safe while detoxing

Who do you call?

Physician

If the patient becomes violent, overly agitated or is a possible danger to self, call security.

You need to know:

- Alcohol withdrawal is common in the hospital
- Alcohol withdrawal can be fatal if not treated properly
- These patients are at increased risk for seizures
- The nursing staff needs to closely monitor vital signs and CIWA-Ar scores
- Most hospital policies and procedures state that if a person's CIWA score is above 15, then the patient should be transferred to the ICU.
- Labs and electrolytes need to be monitored closely
- It is usually a good idea to get a chest x-ray and an EKG
- ETOH withdrawal protocols are based on the patient's signs and symptoms.

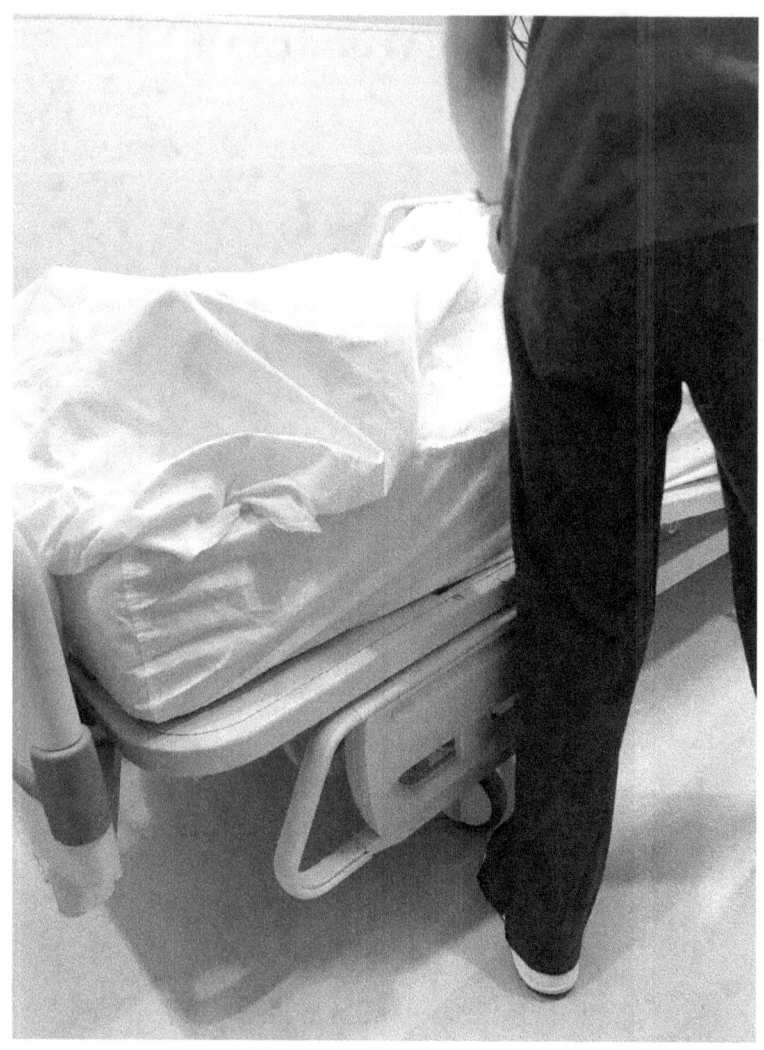

The physician may order:

- CIWA protocol which usually includes
  - Vitamins
  - Labs
  - Benzodiazepines (usually Ativan)
  - Vitamins including folic acid
  - Labs

- Electrolyte monitoring
- EKG
- CXR
- Famotidine

Points to Remember:

- Do not judge the patient
- Alcohol withdrawal symptoms can happen in any age group. It does not discriminate.
- Symptoms can sometimes be unpredictable. They are not on a time schedule.
- As the acute care nurse, you are responsible for keeping the patient and the staff safe. Do not take this responsibility lightly.

Because hospital emergencies can happen at any time, it is important to make sure that every patient has a working IV.

Hypoglycemia

Goal:

To get the blood sugar up to an adequate level.

Notes:

Most hospitals have protocols that address the steps to take for hypoglycemia. Hypoglycemia is usually defined as any blood sugar that is below 70.

Hypoglycemia needs to be monitored carefully.

It can happen whether the patient is NPO or eating.

A physician needs to give the hypoglycemic protocol orders to the nurse.

If the patient is symptomatic or if orders are needed STAT, call your charge nurse and the rapid medical team.

If a patient is NPO, on a feeding tube, has a history of hypo/hyperglycemia, or is on an insulin protocol, it is always a good idea to ask the doctor for this protocol to be added. Better safe than sorry.

In some people, the blood glucose levels fall in the middle of the night. It is advised to monitor the levels, especially if HS sliding scale insulin was given.

Severe hypoglycemia can lead to loss of consciousness and seizures. It can be fatal.

Know the signs of mild to moderate hypoglycemia.

See if you can identify the triggering events of the hypoglycemic episode. These may be a delay in a meal,

NPO status, tapering of steroids, HS insulin dose, too aggressive of a sliding scale, introduction of long acting insulin, etc. This will help the physician to correct the issue.

What the protocol usually includes:

If the patient is able to eat/drink, they can be given 15 grams of a carbohydrate. This is usually 8 oz of juice or some milk. Patients can also be given oral glucose.

If the patient is not able to eat or drink, IV dextrose is usually given. Sometimes the facility may also offer glucagon IM, however the go-to is usually IV Dextrose. With IV dextrose, most policies state that the nurse should give half of the amp of D50, retest the blood glucose in 20 minutes and reassess. If the remainder of the dextrose is indicated, then it may be given at this time.

After hypoglycemia is corrected, continue to closely monitor the patient and the glucose levels. Make sure you call the physician and chart what happened.

Review the signs and symptoms of the conditions listed in this book. Take notes on the pages. Remember that this is just a basic outline. Look at your hospital policies and add to each page as indicated.

Learning for nurses never ends.

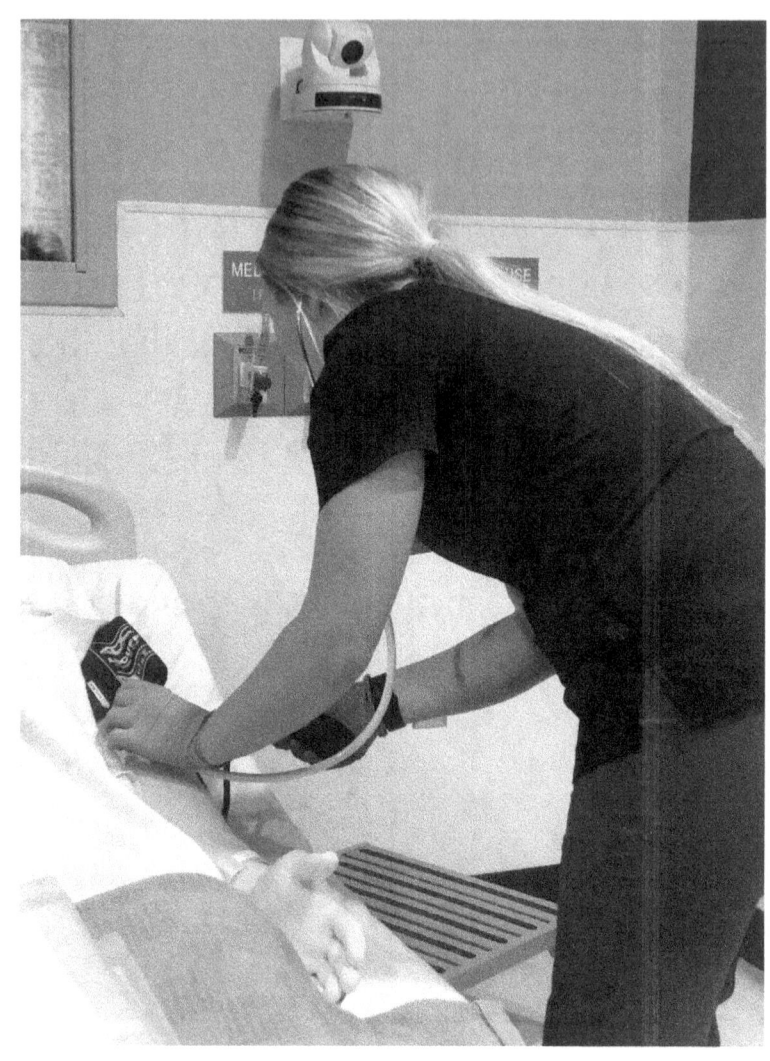

What is a differential diagnosis?

Q: I've heard physicians use the term "differential diagnosis," but I am unsure what it is.

A: When the physicians list a differential diagnosis, that means that they are making a list of possible diseases or conditions that could be causing the symptoms. In order to create a differential diagnosis, the physician needs to put on his/her medical detective hat and collect information. Although medicine is considered a science, it is not always cut and dry.

Physicians often rule out the most serious possible causes (differential diagnosis) first. So if a patient comes in with upper abdominal pain that started suddenly, the physician may feel that it is necessary to rule out a heart issue. I think of the differential diagnosis as a physician brainstorming activity.

Symptoms: It has feathers and a beak.

Differential Diagnosis: Could be a duck, goose, peafowl (not a peacock or a peahen), smaller bird, etc.

More information: It has a large colorful tail.

Differential diagnosis: Peacock, widowbird, Ribbon-tailed Astrapia, Lady Amherst's pheasant, Bird of Paradise.

More Information: It is about 12 pounds.

Physician diagnosis: Peacock

Blood pressure and stroke

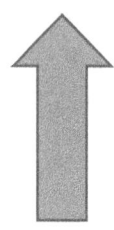 Ischemic CVA, Blood pressure
Is often left higher

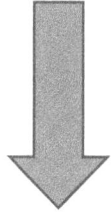 Hemorrhagic CVA, Blood
Pressure is often kept lower.

Code Stroke

Goal:

Minimize damage. Diagnose and treat (if possible), then rehab and prevention.

Things to remember:

- Activate the stroke team, you are on the clock
- NIHSS assessment
- STAT blood glucose
- CT (with/without contrast) STAT (to rule out hemorrhagic stroke)
- MRI/MRA (gold standard to diagnose ischemic stroke)
- Consult neurologist
- Get vitals
- Note time last seen normal- this can help with diagnosis and treatment
- Note TPA exclusions as designated by the American Heart Association. Also remember that the use of TPA is the decision of the physician in charge.
- Labs (INR, PT/aPTT, A1c, ESR, CMP, etc)

Nursing care after the acute phase often includes:

- Patient and family education
  (Most hospitals have stroke information prepared for the patient and family members.)

- Bedside swallow study (if the patient fails the bedside swallow test, then a video swallow test is often ordered).
- Possible head elevation (30 to 45 degrees)
- Speech consult
- PT/OT consult
- Foley
- Rehab consult
- Case management consult
- Monitoring of vital signs (with blood pressure management and temperature control)
- NIHSS on admission and discharge, brief NIHSS q4h
- DVT prophylaxis
- Medications
- Sometimes a psychiatric consultation is also warranted

As you care for the patient, the physicians will try to figure out why the stroke occurred. Was it possibly caused by HTN, a-fib, stimulants, or diabetes? Once the possible cause has been identified, then that course of treatment will begin.

KNOW YOUR HOSPITAL POLICY AS IT PERTAINS TO **CODE STROKE**

GET YOUR NIHSS TRAINING AS SOON AS POSSIBLE. MOST HOSPITALS OFFER IT FREE TO NURSES, HOWEVER IT IS ALSO OFFERED ON-LINE THROUGH THE AMERICAN HEART ASSCIATION-AMERICAN STROKE ASSOCIATION FOR A VERY SMALL FEE.

Code Status

Nurses sometimes have trouble talking about code status with patients, however this is a vital conversation that needs to be done. If you have ever given chest compressions to a person, you will never forget it. The feel of the bones breaking below your hands is an experience like no other. Caring for people after a code is also an experience that few forget. It is a tough reality of nursing.

Once the concept of a code becomes an experience, most nurses feel more comfortable talking about the patient's wishes. If your patient does not want to have CPR performed on them if they should code, then they need to complete a DNR advanced directive. In most hospitals, this can be completed with case management or social work. In most states, it is required to be notarized and the case manager knows all of the notaries in the hospital.

A copy of the advance directive should be kept in the chart.

If the patient plans on being a full code, then there is no problem and nothing needs to be signed.

If nothing is signed, then it should be assumed that the patient is a full code.

What is in a toxicology screen?

When a patient has altered mental status a physician may find that it is necessary to order a toxicology screen (also known as a "tox screen."). Even though a tox screen can be performed through urine, blood, hair, saliva or even sweat, most hospitals use a patient's urine to complete a basic screen. A standard toxicology test screens for:

- Amphetamines
- Barbituates
- Cocaine
- Methamphetamines
- Marijuanna
- Opiates
- Phencyclidine (PCP)

As you can see, there are many drugs that are not included in a basic toxicology screen. It is important to note that just because the toxicology screen comes back negative, it does not mean that the patient did not use another drug. Nurses have to use their gut feeling. If other drugs are suspected, additional tests can be performed, however the treatment is usually the same in that the basic ABC's must be supported.

It is also important to know that local poison centers are always a great source of information for the medical team.

The goal of the emergency department is to stabilize the patient and transfer to either inpatient status or to discharge the patient.

Emergency department nurses are always on the clock. There are often more patients than there is time. Because of this time constraint, the emergency department team performs a focused assessment. They need to treat and admit, or treat and street.

Floor nursing is different than emergency nursing in that assessments must involve the entire patient. When unit nurses get report from the emergency department nurses, they often get frustrated because the report is so targeted to the ailment.

When a patient comes into the emergency department, they do not give the medical team much to go on. They may just tell the staff that they have a stomach pain, or they have a headache. It is up to the staff to get to the bottom of what is really going on. Because the emergency room sees so many patients in a 24 hour period, they just do not have time to complete a full body assessment. It is important for unit nurses to understand this.

Hemothorax

A type of pleural effusion

Often diagnosed with a chest x-ray (CXR).

Usually treated with a chest tube that is inserted in the lower pleural space.

Often hooked up to low intermittent suction (LIS).

If trauma is involved, it is important to note if the patient is taking blood thinning medications.

It is important to monitor the patient, the chest tube site and the atrium.

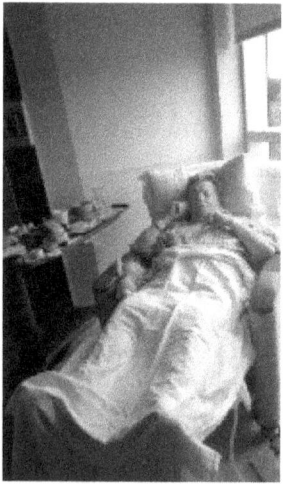

Review what the nurse is supposed to do if the chest tube is dislodged or comes unconnected.

Make sure that the chest tube is only clamped when it is supposed to be.

Know your hospital policies and procedures.

(My mom)

LABS

Basic Metabolic Panel (BMP) vs a Comprehensive Metabolic Panel (CMP)

BMP	CMP
Also known as a "chem-8"	**Also known as a "chem-14"**
Includes:	*Includes:*
Calcium	Albumin
Carbon dioxide	Alkaline phosphatase (ALP)
Chloride	Alanine aminotransferase (ALT)
Creatinine	Aspartate aminotransferase (AST)
Glucose	Blood urea nitrogen (BUN)
Potassium	Calcium
Sodium	Carbon dioxide
Blood urea nitrogen (BUN)	Chloride
	Creatinine
	Glucose
	Potassium
	Sodium
	Total billirubin
	Total protein

*If a chem-8 does not include calcium, then it is called a chem-7.

*Samples are often collected in a light green or dark green lab tube.

LABS

The Complete Blood Count (CBC) vs the Complete Blood Count with Differential

CBC	CBC with diff
White blood cells (WBC)	White blood cells (WBC)
Red blood cells (RBC)	Red blood cells (RBC)
Hemoglobin (Hbg)	Hemoglobin (Hbg)
Hematocrit (Hct)	Hematocrit (Hct)
Mean corpuscular volume (MCV)	Mean corpuscular volume (MCV)
Platelets	Platelets
MCH	MCH
Hemoglobin concentration (MCHC)	Hemoglobin concentration (MCHC)
	Neutrophil
	Lymphocyte
	Monocyte
	Eosinophil
	Basophil

*CBC is often collected in a lavender lab tube

As the nurse, it is your responsibility to make sure that your patient rooms have:

- oxygen, oxygen connectors and tubing
  - Suction supplies
    - Supplies
      - Iv pole
      - Iv pumps
  - SCD machine (unless in the ER)
  - All equipment must be clean and operational.

- It is also your responsibility to make sure that the rooms are clean and without clutter.
- If the patient is considered a fall risk, the bed alarm must be on and fall risk protocol must be in place.
- It is also your responsibility to update the communication board in each of your patient's rooms.

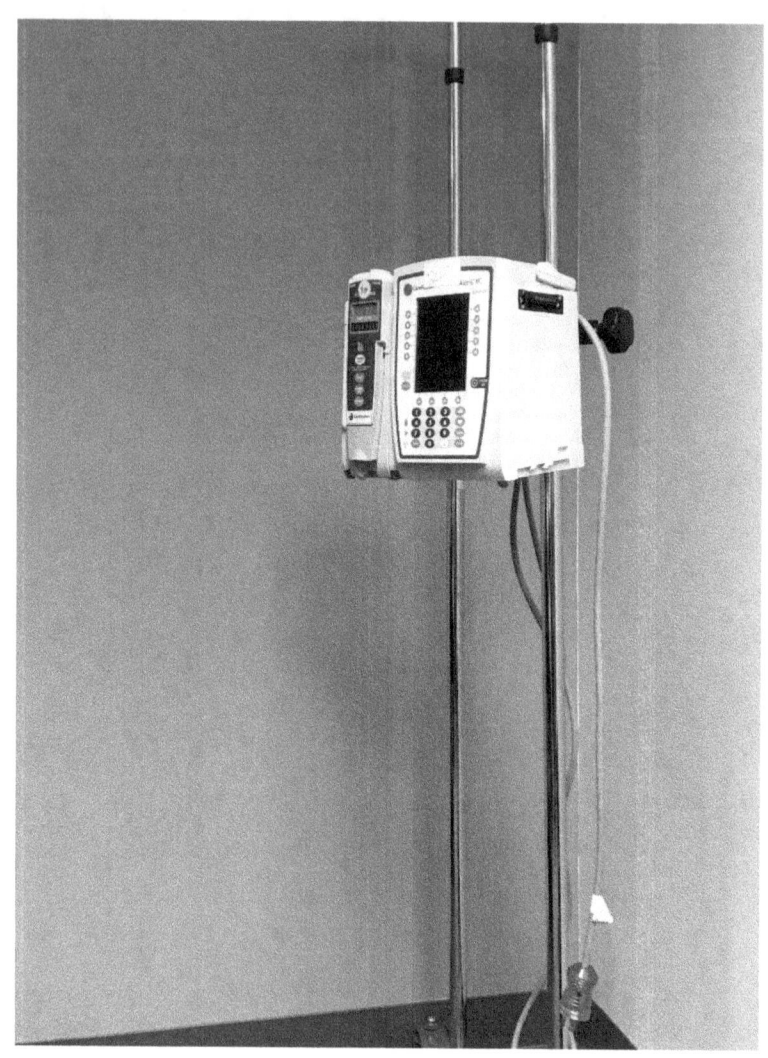

ACLS

Take some time to review the ACLS protocol as indicated by the American Heart Association:

- Bradycardia

- Tachycardia

- PEA
  (Hint: <u>P</u>ush <u>E</u>pi <u>A</u>lways)

- V-tach

- V-fib

- Asystole

- 1st degree heart block

- Second degree heart block, type 1

- Second type heart block, type 2

- 3rd degree heart block

A few ways to remember things:

When I eat M & M's I need to pace myself and eat 2 at a time.

M & M= 2 mg morphine and 2 mg midazolam before pacing.

PEA = Push Epi Always

Asystole: Flat line means compressions in time

Diabetic Ketoacidosis

It is an emergency

Points to remember:

This emergency can occur in people who have been diagnosed with Diabetes type I or Diabetes type II, although I have seen times when the person has not been diagnosed.

Seems to increase with steroid therapy. That is why it is so important to monitor people who are on steroid therapy.

Occurs when a person's body is not producing enough insulin to allow sugar to enter the cells. As a result the body starts to use stored fat to fuel itself, which releases acids called ketones. When these acids build up, it can be fatal.

Signs and symptoms can develop very quickly.

Is more likely to occur when a person is ill or is not using insulin as needed.

Is also more likely to occur when a person has a heart attack, uses drugs/alcohol or has some sort of traumatic event (Mayo Foundation, 1998-2018).

What you will most likely see:

High blood glucose levels that seem to be very resistant to the patient's usual treatments.

Ketones in urine and blood.

Nausea/vomiting, confusion, frequent need to urinate, shortness of breath (breath often smells fruity), abdominal pain.

Common Steps in Hospital Treatment

Labs usually include: UA, serum ketones, CBC w/ diff, Lactate, Magnesium, CMP

May also need blood cultures, ABG's, troponin

Consult Endocrinology Physician STAT

Fluid bolus

Insulin drip w/ frequent glucose checks

Electrolyte monitoring and correction (especially potassium)

Watch serum bicarb (CO_2)

EKG

Chest x-ray

Admit or transfer to the ICU

Mayo Foundation (1998-2018). Diabetic ketoacidosis. Retrieved from www.mayoclinic.org.

Nurse-to-Nurse Report

In order for nurse-to-nurse reports to be the most efficient, a methodical method must be established.

Basic Information is first:

Patient name, room number, date of birth, code status, isolations status, allergies

Admitting and consulted physicians

Where did the patient come from (home, SNF, be specific if possible)?

Why are they here?

Background information on what happened (condensed version).

What have we done or are planning to do for the primary issue? Review results if actions are complete.

Review brief medical history.

Current Assessment:

Neuro (include Psych)

- Alert and oriented?
- NIH?
- ETOH withdrawal?
- HOH?
- Sight issues?
- Ambulation

Cardiovascular

- Rhythm
- Rate

- Pulses
- Paced
- LCEF (if known)
- Last blood pressure

Respiratory

- SAT
- O2? Vent? Trach?
  - **If on a ventilator- include the settings, trach type and size, inline suctioning, etc.**
  - Does the patient wear O2 at home?
  - Is it a new trach?
- Sleep Apnea (wear CPAP @ night?), Do they have their home one? Is RT managing it?
- Lung Sounds
- Receiving RT treatments?

GI/GU

- Does the patient have a urine catheter? Is the urine catheter present or removed? If removed, when?
- Incontinent?
- Last time urinated? Color? Any issues?
- Was a UA sent?
- Last BM? Any problems?
- Does the patient have a rectal tube?

IV

- IV? PICC? Midline?
  - Where?
  - When placed?
  - Gauge?
  - Size?
  - Any problems?

Skin

- Any issues or problems?
- Any pressure sores?
- What are we doing for issues?
- Last bath/oral care

ACHS/Q6H glucose checks?

- Does the patient have diabetes?
- Are they on steroids?
- Sliding scale?
- What type?

Tests/labs/procedures

- Is the patient on electrolyte replacement protocol?
- Any labs we are concerned about?
- Upcoming draws?

Plan

- Discharge planning?
- Needed patient educated?
- What do I need to do this shift?

Ask if the nurse has any questions.

Once you practice the flow of the report, you will be able to organize your thoughts and information in a standard way. Practice giving report like this. Your fellow nurses will be grateful.

If you can organize your report sheet in this manner, it will help you give reports.

SBAR's MADE SIMPLE

(AND CHANGING THEM TO SBART's)

When you call a doctor, there just isn't a lot of time. They do not have time to waste and you do not have time to waste. SBAR was created to keep things simple and communication streamlined.

S	Introduce yourself, what unit. Patient name and room number. Who is the primary doctor from the practice? State the problem.	*Hi Dr. Smith, this is Anne from CCU. I am taking care of Dr. Jone's patient Patty Patient in room 300. She is currently c/o 8/10 abdominal pains. The pains are not radiating and occurred after she ate dinner. This is new for her.*
B	Why was pt. admitted? Treatment for the problem to date. Any pertinent background/medical history.	*She was admitted with pneumonia. She has no known GI issues that we are aware of.*
A	Last vital signs (if appropriate) on O2? Any changes in last assessment?	*Her current blood pressure is 150/75, pulse is 60, RR 18, O2 SAT is 98% on room air, temp 98.1. She states that she has not had a bowel movement for 3 days, which is not normal for her.*

R	What do you recommend? You are the one with the patient. It is okay if you don't know what to do. Ask them what they recommend? Ask if they want any tests, labs, medications given. READ BACK THE ORDERS TO MAKE SURE THAT YOU HAVE THEM RIGHT.	*Do you think that we should get an abdominal x-ray? Are there any other tests that you want? Should I order any labs? She is currently only scheduled for a BMP in the morning. Can I give her something for the pain? Are there any other medications that you would like me to order?*
T	Thank them for their time. Tell them that you will keep them posted.	*Thank you Dr. Smith. I will keep you posted with any changes.*

S= Situation

B= background

A= Assessment

R= Recommendations

T= Thank them

**It is important to document in the chart every time you talk to a physician.

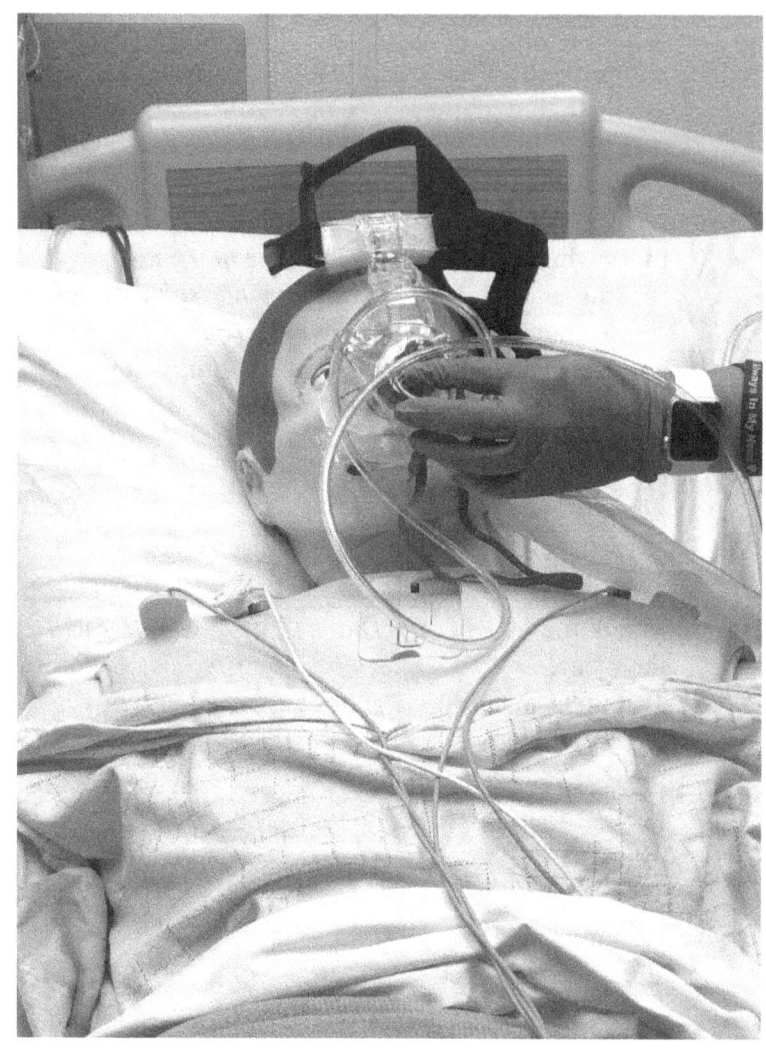

Personal Motto:
"I will be the best nurse that I can be."

Self- Learning

Take some time to learn about:
- o Pacemakers
- o ICD's
- o Cardiac Procedures
  - o Stent placement
  - o ECHO's
  - o Stress tests
- o Cardiac Rehabilitation
- o Ventilators
- o Labs

Make sure you:
- o Invest in your business
  - o Become certified
  - o Take continuing education classes online and in person
  - o Network
  - o Create a website for you
  - o Join professional organizations
  - o Float to other units and learn

I hope that you enjoy this book. I write all of my books with love. I want to help other nurses learn the basics and I am dedicated to nurse empowerment. Never be afraid to ask questions. We never know everything.

I will try to continue to update the information in this book as practice changes. Please remember that the recipes in this book are just basics. They are not recommendations.

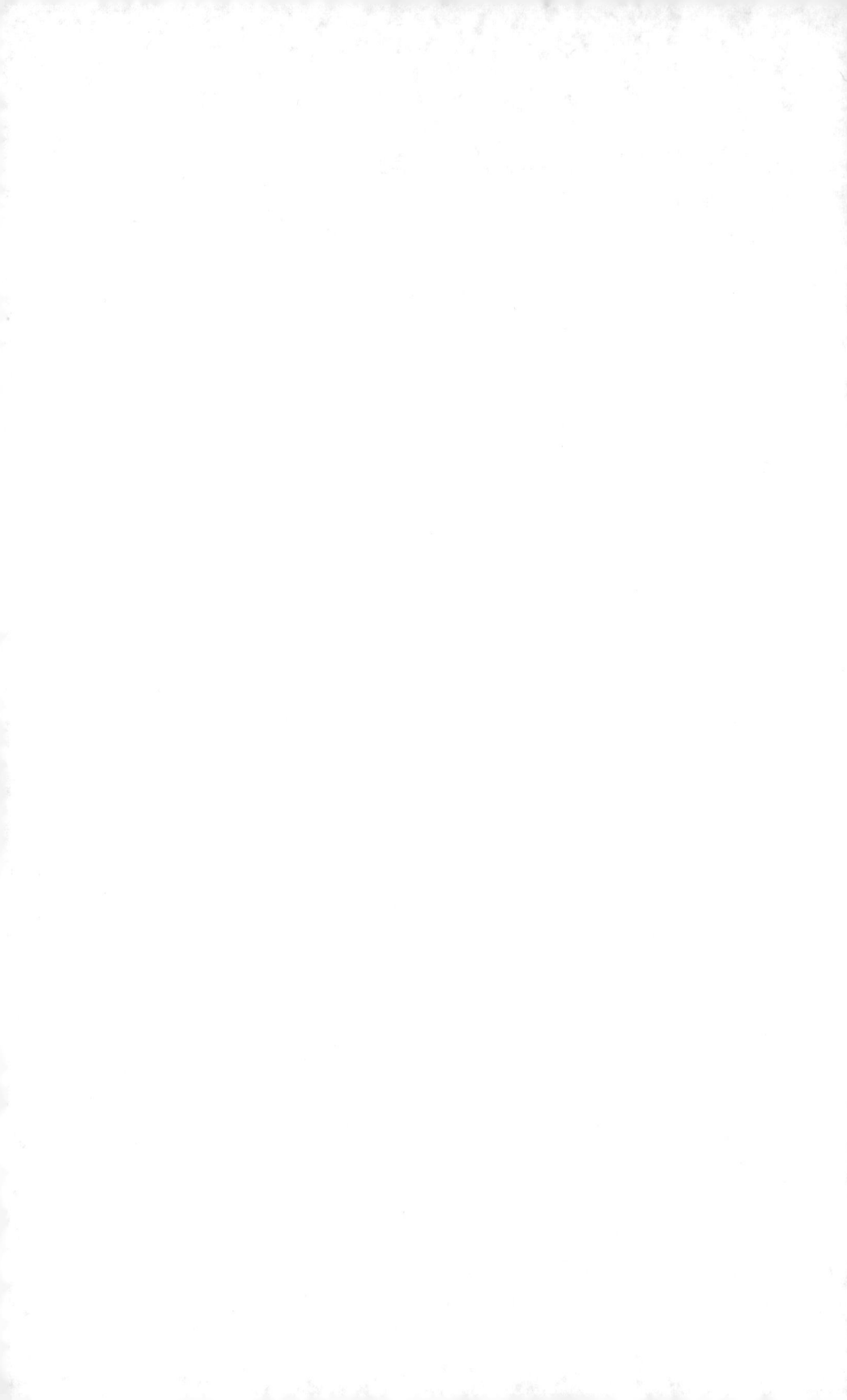